There's No Exercise Like Morning

Exercise for a Healthy Mind and Body

The Health Buff

MP Publishing

Copyright

Table of Contents

INTRODUCTION

It is not just conventional wisdom that morning exercise works best for us in terms of rejuvenating us both mentally physically. This is something that many fitness specialists will tell you. Above all, your body tells you that. It is a no brainer that any activity we perform after a restful night's sleep will be at a higher level of efficiency than any other time of the day. As in most cases, if it feels good, it usually is good for you.

It is, however, heartening to know that science backs our bodily instinct. A study carried out by the Appalachian State University discovered that people who exercised at 7 am produced a larger quantity of Human Growth Hormone (HGH) than those who exercised much later. Besides, they would go to sleep faster at night. In particular our testosterone levels are more than 30% higher in the mornings, making us more energetic, and allowing for greater muscle development. No wonder most people find exercising in the morning so much more fun.

However, not all of us are morning people. The very thought of waking up at the crack of dawn and heading for the gym gives quite a few people the shivers. But there are people out there who are perfectly happy doing that and heartily recommend it to whosoever would care to listen.

Why do they do that? What do they know that the one's who are quite content to roll out of bed only after the sun is blazing with a fair bit of intensity do not? If you are one of those who think that way, then reading this book will not just shake you out of your complacency, but also have you get up at the crack of dawn and have a go at metamorphosing yourself.

Chapter 1

Morning Makeover

Most of us would want to better our lives, irrespective of whether we are comfortably placed in life or struggling to make a mark. This implies that the instinct of wanting to do better than we are, exists in everyone. It is hardwired into our brain. Yet many of us, let time and opportunity slip us by. We forget both that we all possess the mettle to strive and improve ourselves and the fact that time once lost, never comes back.

Finding the motivation to exercise in the morning comes from realizing the immense benefits that come your way by doing so. In the main these are-

1.   Improved Metabolism- The great thing about a workout is that the human bodies burn more calories after completing one than during it. It has been found out that people who exercise, burn an

additional 190 calories in the fourteen hours following the exercise regime than those who do not.

This means that if your morning begins with a workout, you have set yourself up for a full day of burning calories, even while you go about your routine daily activities. Because exercising early in the morning raises your rate of metabolism, whatever you subsequently eat during the day gets utilized in providing nourishment to your charged up body, rather than getting stored as fat. The result is a leaner, fitter and healthier you.

2. Enhanced Physical and Mental Well-Being- Instead of reaching for your caffeine fix early in the morning to energize yourself for the day ahead, it is a much better idea to work out some sweat exercising. Not only does that invigorate you physically for the day ahead, but it also makes you mentally sharp and alert with a much improved focus. It is estimated that even a short early morning workout has twice the impact that a cup of coffee has in freshening up and energizing the human mind.

3. Better Sleep- If you follow a daily routine of getting up early in the morning and exercising, there is no question about the fact that you will get a good night's sleep. For all the stresses of modern day life, a simple early morning exercise ritual will ensure that you both get the energy to go through the day with vigor, but also manage to get your desired quota of sleep every night.

You will not get the same impact if you exercise in the afternoon or the evening. The simple reason for this is that exercise cranks up the metabolism rate, which is not at all conducive to sleeping. You want a night of restful sleep, make sure that you exercise early in the morning.

4. Enhanced Self-Discipline- While it is all very well to want to exercise early in the morning to reap its many benefits, the fact of the matter is that it requires a great deal of discipline to do that. So many of us start on an exercise regime with great enthusiasm, but soon find ourselves slacking.

This is especially true of an early morning exercise regime. Being able to stick to an exercise schedule that would have you get up early in the morning every day and sweat it out, definitely requires iron-clad discipline. Therefore, the very act of waking up early, day after day after day and faithfully following a prescribed exercise routine, enhances your self discipline substantially. This is something that will benefit you in every aspect of your life.

5.   Better Quality Of Life- Beginning your day with exercise sets the tone for a great day ahead. You feel in top shape physically as well as mentally to take on the rigors of the day and when night falls you are ready to get your nightly quota of restful sleep.

With time your overall quality of life will take on another dimension. Regular exercise is known to cure everything from the common cold to indigestion to depression. Regular exercise helps the body release endorphins- the happiness hormones. You truly will live a truly enjoyable life.

Chapter 2

The Science Behind Morning Exercise

While we all instinctively know that exercising in the morning works wonderfully well in keeping our bodies and minds,in fine fettle, what does science have to say? Apparently pretty much the same thing. A part of the reason why early morning workouts are more efficient at promoting wellbeing has to do with the practicality of it.

If you follow an early morning exercise schedule, there are greater chances of your sticking to it. Workouts scheduled later in the day, often don't occur because one's daily routine more often than not gets disturbed due to some reason or the other-unscheduled meetings, getting stuck in the traffic, so on and so forth. The biggest impediment to exercising early in the morning is the motivation to make the effort.

Who would like to leave the snug comfort of one's bed early in the morning? But if you have compelling reasons backed by science to encourage you to do the right thing, you most likely would. Here's what these reasons are-

1.   Fat Loss- We all love that one. Exercise to lose fat! But how often does that happen or how well does that happen. Not very, right? The reason probably lies in the fact that they are probably exercising at the wrong time of the day. There is credible research that suggests that early morning exercise prior to having breakfast causes fat oxidation.

     Besides, you will not put on fat, even if you have a colorie-rich diet post morning exercised undertaken in an empty stomach.

2.   Enhanced Testosterone Levels- Early morning is when the testosterone levels peak, which enables you to give your workout its all. That apart, you are able to build extra muscle mass, even while your burn extra calories and lose weight faster. It makes sense to take advantage of the body's

physiology and start early to get maximum leverage from exercise.

In business terms, you get the best ROI (Return On Investment) by exercising in the morning. So why not make the most of it?

3. Better Stress Management- Stress is the bane of modern living. The best way to deal with it is first thing in the morning with a vigorous workout. This helps release endorphins, the mood enhancing hormones giving you a good start to your day.

   If you make this a daily routine, you will have found a great way to reduce your daily stress levels, leading to a more productive and happier life.

4. Early Morning Exercise Makes You Consume Fewer Calories- Now here's an interesting piece of information about the benefits of early morning exercise. According to research carried out by researchers from Brigham Young University early morning exercise leads to a decrease in appetite. What's especially heartening to those

trying to lose weight this feeling of wanting to eat less persisted through the day.

This finding is significant in that there are a large number of people who exercise quite a bit, but are unable to lose weight because they just can't seem to be eat less. All that such people need do is to schedule their exercise routine in the mornings and weight loss won't be an issue for them anymore.

5.   Reduced Blood Pressure- Exercising early in the morning reduces one's blood pressure by 10% and stays that way through the day. What's more it goes down by as much as 25% at night.

A daily routine of early morning exercise therefore can lead to better heart health, due to a healthier rate of blood-pressure.

6.   Protection Against Diabetes- If one exercises early in the morning prior to having breakfast protects one against both insulin resistance and glucose intolerance, thereby offering protection against Type2 diabetes.

Chapter 3

The Best Morning Exercises

We all know that getting yourself in the mood to exercise soon after you get up in the morning requires a certain level of dedication and motivation. Rather than forcing yourself into performing all manner of complicated exercise routines first thing in the morning, you should figure out what works out best for you. The idea is to stay the course and not carry out a flurry of activity for a few days and then just as quickly give it up.

There are in the main two types of exercises that you need to make a part of your daily morning morning routine. These are-

1.   Simple Body Weight Exercises- This is for those who find it difficult to dedicate a fair amount of time to a vigorous workout in the morning on a

daily basis. Simple exercises that leverage the weight of the body are a quick and efficient way of improving blood circulation, energizing both muscle and mind, tuning the metabolism and burning a few calories

Among the several exercises one can look at performing are sets of push-ups, overhead lunges and squats. One should look at at least two sets of 10 repetitions of the above exercises.

2. Cardio Exercises- Early morning cardiovascular exercises are particularly effective for weight loss. This is because, it stimulates the burning of calorie at a time of the day when the carbohydrate reserves are at the lowest on account of not eating through the night. Of course, the important caveat is that you perform these exercises prior to having breakfast.

If you are not inclined to dedicate a lot of time to do this, the good news is that even a light 30 minute session is quite beneficial. A light half an hour jog in the neighborhood park, just before you tuck into your breakfast would suffice quite nicely.

It really is not all that difficult to form a daily routine of early morning exercise, once you realize that you can start by making a modest beginning. Once you start noticing the impact of even thirty minutes of light early morning exercise in tuning your body and improving your mood, you can likely find the motivation to spend a greater amount of time exercising in the morning.

The more you exercise, the greater will be the benefit that will accrue to you. The more involved that you will get in the realm of exercise and fitness, the more you will discover about your own body and mind. You will for instance be amazed to know how resilient nature has made our bodies, and how powerful your mind is.

You can achieve things with your body and mind that you cannot imagine are possible. But for that you truly need to understand the whole science behind exercise, especially early morning exercise. Let us now get you're a little deeper into the fascinating word of morning exercise by telling you about all the major types of exercises you can perform in the morning.

1.   Running or Jogging- This is the most natural of exercises, requiring no training or equipment, save a good pair of running shoes. You could run on a treadmill or out in the open if you like communing with nature. The benefits of running come in the shape of improving the performance of your brain, lifting your mood, reduction in high blood pressure and the incidence of heart disease and an overall increase in life span.

Nature has equipped the human body to run and by not utilizing that faculty, we are doing ourselves the greatest possible disservice. You would be amazed to know that no animal, not even the horse can match us humans in long distance endurance running. With a body built like that, why wouldn't you run? Why wouldn't anyone run? It will cost you nothing, while opening up a whole new world of health and well-being.

2.   Cycling- Cycling is a fantastic cardio exercise that helps burn lots of calories. Again the choice is between cycling indoors in a gym or doing it in

the great outdoors. The only cost that you entail in cycling is a one time investment in the bike itself. Considering the sheer range of benefits that accrue from cycling that is a cost that you might not worry too much about incurring. These include-enhanced muscle strength and flexibility, better mobility of joints, improved posture, stronger bones, reduced fat, disease prevention and so on. If there is a good start to a morning, it surely has to be this!

3. Circuit Training- This all in one fitness routine early in the morning fits in perfectly with today's fast paced lifestyles. Comprising of a series of fast paced exercises its basic premise is to alternate between aerobic exercises like stepping or pedaling away intensely on a stationary cycle with working out with the help of weight machines.

The fact that this form of training both enhances your strength and improves your aerobic fitness while helping you burn a good number of calories early in the morning, makes it one comprehensive routine that you would do well to adopt.

4. Stretching Exercises- You should certainly look at incorporating stretching exercises in your daily exercise routine. These exercises help in toning your muscles, imparting spinal flexibility and preventing arthritis.

These exercises also warm you up for a more vigorous routine. Besides, your posture too improves on account of stretching. A lot of us have desk jobs that require us to sit hunched in front of computers. This tightens our chest muscles and strains are back ones. A morning exercise schedule that includes stretching helps loosen these muscles. Stretching also helps remove muscular and joint pain. That apart, it increases blood flow to the body, while also energizing you for the day ahead.

5. Push Ups- We all know what push ups are, right? It is the exercise where you lie inches from the ground face downward, balancing your body weight on your knees and toes, even while you try to raise and lower yourself as many times as you can

This is a great exercise for strengthening a whole lot of muscle groups, particularly in the chest shoulder and triceps area. In any case, anyone who manages a few sets of pushups in the morning will inevitably feel a rush of energy at the end of the day.

6.   Bicycle Crunches- This exercise that has you lying on your back, bending your knees and trying to alternately make your right elbow touch your left knee your left elbow touch your right knee. This will not only put you in the right mood early in the morning, but also help you keep your weight in check and keep insomnia at bay.

7.   Early Morning Kick Boxing- This is a high-energy workout that is sure to liven up your mornings. What's more, it is a great way of toning your muscles and imparting great flexibility to the body. That apart, it improves blood circulation, helps relieve stress, burns body fat and teaches you a vital art of self-defense.

8. Early Morning Yoga- The Indians perfected the yogic system of exercises over millennia and today the world swears by this holistic system of exercise. Performing yogic exercises first thing in the morning is the best way to put body and soul in perfect harmony with nature.

Among the most energizing of early morning yogic exercises has to be the surya namaskar or salutations to the sun. The surya namaskar process involves a set of salutations that The surya namaskar works by stimulating the solar plexus area with the energy of the early morning sun. Depending upon the speed with which you perform these sets of exercises you could get different types of results. Doing it at a gentle place will impart flexibility to the body, doing it at a medium pace will make the body tones and doing it at a brisk pace will improve as a cardiovascular system and also help one lose weight. Above all, it keeps wards of diseases and keeps you in the pink of health-mentally and physically. As a matter of fact, it will impart a glow to your face. You will not only feel healthy, but look healthy as well.

9.   Morning Walk- This is probably the easiest morning exercise anyone can perform and comes loaded with benefits. Walking first thing in the morning helps in awakening the body the most natural way. By increasing our pulse rate and working up a sweat, we up our level of alertness and feel a definite improvement of mood.

A brisk morning walk moves us from a level of inactivity to one of high energy. Moreover, your blood circulation and hormonal balance too improve and you feel energized for the day ahead. Besides, it's a great way to shed those extra pounds. Perhaps the greatest benefit of an early morning exercise is the fact that it is good for your heart. People who walk in the mornings on a consistent basis at a speed of 3 to 4 miles an hour reduce their chances of having a heart attack by about 40%. Other benefits include an enhanced social life in the shape of your morning walk companion or companions and the fact that it gives you the time to chalk out your program for the day ahead.

10.	Swimming- You may think that swimming is an afternoon activity, but think again. But imagine coinciding your swim with the rising sun. An early morning way is one of the easiest ways to give yourself a comprehensive early morning workout. It is especially beneficial to people suffering from joint pain as swimming allows one to move without causing much stress to the body. The biggest advantage of an early morning swim is the fact that it boosts your metabolism at the right time. Consequently, you burn calories through the day. Another advantage of an early morning swim is getting exposed to the sifter rays of an early morning sun. While this is gentle on your skin, it provides you with the essential vitamin D.

11.	Early Morning Gymming- The thing about going to a gym in the morning is that it first of al extracts a firm commitment from you toward achieving your fitness with seriousness. Of all forms of exercise, working out in a gym is the most scientifically planned and regulated one. The access to exercise machines and the personal advice of the coaches lets you set high standards for personal fitness for yourself.

What's more, you will even be able to track your progress and see how well you have done. Morning workouts at the gym work quite well for those who are trying to lose weight, because your body will end up using fat, to sustain your early morning workout. It will also leave you feeling fresh for the rest of the day, though initially it might take a little getting used to.

Chapter 4

Precautions To Be Taken During Early Morning Exercise

While there is no doubting the fact that morning exercise is a great way to keep your body and mind in great shape, the fact of the matter is that we need to plan for it. We can't just rush into early morning exercise without taking the due precautions necessary to prevent injury. Given below are tips that will help you plan your daily morning exercise routine in a safe and fruitful way-

1. Go To Bed Early- This is the most important one. If you are planning on an early morning workout, ensure that you go to bed early so as to wake up rested and ready. You will end up harming yourself, if you workout first thing in the morning without providing your body the minimum

amount of sleep it needs to shake off the previous day's tiredness.

2. Warm Up- Don't plunge into a vigorous exercise routine when you start out in the morning. You need to gently warm up your body to prepare it for the rigors of a workout.

Your body temperature is lower than usual when you wake up in the morning and it is therefore unwise to rush things. As you start the process of exercising, your body experiences change in the shape of enhanced blood flow and an increase in the rate of respiration. In order for your body to adjust to these changes a warm up is essential.

3. Don't Go Gymming On An Empty Stomach- If hitting the gym is your idea of a morning workout, then you better not do it on an empty stomach. You will need the energy that is necessary to engage in. It would make sense to consume something like a handful of nuts or fruit a 30 minutes before you start working out at the gym. This will provide you with the right kind of

energy boost to efficiently go through your myriad exercise routines.

4.   No Painkillers- It is a bad idea to exercise after you have had painkillers. The thing is that pain killers relax muscles and that means that you might injure yourself performing some of the resistance and weight exercises. If you have to work out, you could maybe try walking a little.

5.   Boost Your Activity Level Gradually- If you are just starting out with morning exercise, take care to boost your activity level gradually. This will help your body acclimatize itself to the new routine in its own time. You can't be looking at vigorous workouts, the very first day you start your morning exercise routine.

6.   Wear Appropriate Arrire- This is important so that you feel a sense of comfort early in the morning, setting the tone for the day. Be careful about the kind of shoes you are wearing, as these tend to wear out pretty fast during the course of

exercising. Try and change them every six moths or so.

7.   Protects Against Cold- Mornings are cooler than the rest of the day, in all seasons and in winters it can get positively cold in the mornings. It therefore makes sense to protect yourself against cold weather by wearing appropriate clothing. You may want to wear layers clothing and protect your hands by wearing gloves in really cold weather.

If you perform a workout in really cold weather without adequate protection you risk hypothermia. Adequate protection against cold is therefore a must.

Chapter 5

Morning Exercise VS. Evening Exercise

Not everyone is a votary of morning exercises. Some seem to prefer evening exercises. It is not even as if evening exercise won't benefit you. They will. Exercise benefits you whenever you do them. But there is an optimal way of exercising and a sub-optimal way of doing it.

As to which time is best suited for exercise, it depends upon the type of exercise you are undertaking, what you aim to achieve with it, the weather conditions, the physiology of your body and so on. That withstanding both exercising in the morning and evening have distinct advantages. Lets see how these two stack up against each other.

Morning Exercise- There are a large number of people who sincerely believe that mornings are the best time to be exercising. The body is rested and the mind is fresh and what better time than that to perform exercises. Then there are those who can't bear the thought to put their bodies through the rigors of exercise first thing in the morning and think evenings are the best time for exercising.

That being stated, you cannot also doubt the wisdom of the many who swear that morning exercise positively rocks. A study carried out by the University of New South Wales found out that exercising in the morning , prior to having breakfast is the ideal time for performing cardio exercises with the intention of losing weight.

This is on account of your body having to burn fat, stored in the body on account of your having used up your store of glycogen during the hours you would have slept at night. That apart, exercising in the morning gives a fillip to your body's rate of metabolism, keeping you alert and active during the course of the day.

Another study carried out by the University of Glasgow found out that morning exercises boosts a person's mood, more than exercising in the evening does. This is on account of the fact that exercising in the morning helps the body release the feel-good endorphins, thereby elevating our mood ad imparting s sense of well being. To cap it all, exercising in the morning allows you to sleep well at night, enabling you to get up fresh and raring to start your morning exercise routine

Evening Exercise

While morning exercise, certainly has its advantages, evening exercise score when it comes to sheer performance evening times are better for exercising. In fact, a study published in published in Sport's Medicine magazine supported the contention that performance was better when one exercised in the evening.

Late evening is ideal for performing the kind of exercises that aid in muscle build-up. That means high intensity exercises, such as weight training are better performed in the evening when the muscles are already warmed up and more amenable to for an extended workout. The higher level of testosterone present in the body in the latter part of the day, also make it easier to perform intense muscle building exercises in the evening.

Besides, you will no longer have to stress about having to prepare to wake up early in the morning, and starting your exercise routine. Instead, you can go to bed without a care in this regard and wake up at a decent hour the next morning. Another perk of an evening workout is the fact that one will be able to relieve oneself of all the accumulated stresses of the day.

As to which of the two methods of exercising is better, it really depends upon what you expect from your daily workout. If holistic good health encompassing a healthy mind and body is what your primary aim is behind daily exercise, then morning exercise is a better bet for you. If getting beefed up and increasing muscle volume and strength is what you are looking at, then exercising in the evening is definitely for you.

In the ultimate analysis, it is your overall wellbeing, rather than the size and shape of your muscles that should matter. So, in the balance we could possibly say that exercising in the mornings is probably the better option of the two.

Chapter 6

Motivating Yourself to Exercise in The Morning

Well begun they say is half done. That is certainly true of exercising in the morning. Despite knowing about its myriad positive effects in imparting upon us the gifts of a healthy body and mind, quite a large number of us just can't seem to muster the will to commit to a daily routine of early morning exercise.

It is almost as if a primeval force is stopping us from doing so. Do you remember how as a small child, you just hated to leave the warm comfort of your bed and head to school? Often, your parents had to literally drag you out of bed and pack you off to school. But as you grew older, there came a day, when you actually looked forward to go to school where you could catch up with your buddies, participate in the sports played there, and make plans for your future academic career. You had come to realize that your school was the crucible where your destiny was going to be forged and you were ready to meet the challenge head on.

A somewhat similar trajectory is to be followed in your graduating from being a slacker who does not want to make the effort required for early morning exercise to someone who knows that it is good for you and looks forward to it every morning. This will happen only if you have a good talk with yourself and realize that you need to display a modicum of maturity in accepting that the benefits of an early morning exercise routine, far outweigh its negatives. And what are the negatives really? Your having to discipline yourself to make a commitment to your own well being?Come to think of it, it really is ridiculous to exhibit a school-kid kind of petulance toward your own well being.

However, attractive as the logic of disciplining your own self for your own benefit sounds, we are human at the end of the day, and don't necessarily always do what is in our own best interest. This is as true of eating, as it is of early morning exercise. We know that fruit and vegetables are good for us, but what do we gorge ourselves on? Steaks, pizzas and burgers!

It would almost seem that we are addicted to self-harm. While that is not really true, we often struggle with motivating ourselves to achieve something worthwhile. That being stated we can take a few simple steps that can help us overcome inertia and get into the wholesome routine of early morning exercising.

1. Rope in a partner- Humans are a social species of animal, and dont really excel at doing things alone. Even Robinson Cruisoe truly came into his own after Man Friday came into his life. So get yourself a partner in crime, an exercise partner to be more precise. It could be a family member or a friend who lives nearby.

    The ideal partner would be someone who shares your fitness goals and wouldn't mind getting up early in the morning along with you and exercising. If your partner resents having to do so and is constantly cribbing, you won't really be going very far with your morning exercise goals.

With a motivated partner on the other hand, you could push each other to improve upon your performance. If one of you feels low the other could pep you up and you could do so on his low days. Besides, a healthy competition between the two of you will motivate you to put in your best effort.

2.   Set Yourself A Fitness Goal- If we have a coveted target to achieve like fitting into a favorite t-shirt and jeans that we have long outgrown, we will likely push ourselves to lose weight, come what may. Even if this means getting up at the crack of dawn and going for a long jog.

It might not be a bad idea to prominently display the object of your focus to stop you from wavering in your pursuit of the goals. In the above case, hanging the clothing in your closet in a manner that you see it every day might do the trick.

3.   Sleep Well and Well In Time- Nothing like a bad night's sleep to dampen one's enthusiasm for early morning exercise. You should go to bed

early to be fit for early morning exercising the next day. A minimum of seven to eight hours sleep is a must.

If you sleep less than that your body will produce the appetite enhancing hormone that will send your diet for a toss and negate the gains of any exercising you might have done.

4.	Use a funky alarm-message- This is one of the perks of the digital age. Record yourself a wake up message that really inspires you- anything from a drill sergeant's yell to birds chirping mellifluously.

5.	Socialize at the gym- The gym is a great place to make friends with like minded people who share your fitness goals. Bonding with them every morning will make you part of a small community who will lookout for each other.

6.	Schedule a daily morning workout-Many of us often forget all the important things we need to do unless we formally schedule them. With so much competing for our attention, what with work and personal commitments taking up most of our times, it is way too easy to forget one's early morning exercise routine.

So it makes eminent sense to create a weekly exercise schedule at the start of every week. This could for example be spending an hour in the gym every morning before leaving for work, Monday to Friday or it could comprise of an hour of jogging every morning prior to breakfast, five days a week.

Once you commit in writing a schedule, you will discover that there is a greater chance of your sticking to it. In case you skip a day's scheduled workout, right down the reason for it. You will discover that more often than not it is an excuse for not exercising. By writing it down, you may be compelled to stp making them.

7.   Use Workout Music- Music is a tremendous mood-lifter. If you have a peppy playlist on your i-Pod or mobile phone, you will want to work out every morning. Anyone who has exercised while listening to music will agree that it enhances your ability to work out much harder than you normally

would. Upbeat peppy music is a great fatigue buster. Why do you think that the armies of the world have such marvelous bands that belt out the most upbeat marching tunes?

8.   Give Yourself A Reward- If you have been a good girl or a good boy and managed to achieve a fitness milestone by scrupulously sticking to a morning exercise schedule reward yourself. Maybe you could buy yourself another one of that pair of jeans that you can now easily manage to fit into. Or maybe you and your exercise could go watch an NBC game at the basketball stadium with the exercise buddy who helped you achieve your fitness goal.

9.   Share Your Morning Workout Routine On Social Media- This is a great way of letting the world know how serious you are about your fitness routine and what you have achieved today. With apps and trackers providing you with precise data of how much you have achieved in your morning workout, go ahead and post it on Facebook , Twitter, Insatagram and so on.

Chapter 7

Celebrities Who Exercise In The Mornings

Most of us look up to celebrities and part of the reason has to do with their looking like gods and goddesses. All the time! How do they do it? By exercising and eating right of course! You can do the same. Do you know how many of the celebrities you so admire work out in the mornings? A very large number of them. Here's the lowdown.

1. President Barak Obama- When he was President, Obama would start his very busy day with a 6:45 am workout. Imagine! Would there be a man who would be busier and more harried than the President of the United States? Yet he found the

time to exercise in the morning. What makes you think that you have a busier schedule than that?

2. Dwayne Johnson- Who else? Dwayne Johnson A.K.A, The Rock swears by his morning workout. He is up and about at 4.45 am going through his exercise routine. Now do you believe that early morning workouts are nothing short of AWESOME!

3. Steve Reinmund, former Chairman and CEO, Pepsi-This highly successful corporate executive, who is now the dean of a business school starts his day with a 5 am four mile run. This, when he is a father of teenage children with a host of duties and responsibilities. If he can make time for early morning exercising, then why shouldn't you be able to.

4. Michelle Gass, President, Starbucks- While she may be making coffee popular in the world, her own early morning stimulation comes from from her early morning 4:30 am run. She has been doing this for a decade and a half credits her

morning workout with the success she has achieved in life.

5. Anna Wintour, Editor-in-chief, Vogue-This inspirational figure whom the world admires wakes up before its dawn and works out by playing an hour of tennis. Somehow there is some kind of a special gift that iconic figures have about working out around the time of dawn.

6. Kevin O' Leary, Chairman O' Leary- His day starts at 5.30 am when he checks out the international bond market following which he cycles for 45 minutes, while watching TV. Not a moment to spare, but still enough time to exercise.

7. Oprah Winfrey, Media Mogul-Like in the case of other successful women, her day begins pretty early too. In her case her wellness routine comprises of meditation and a treadmill workout.

8. Bill Gates, Founder, Microsoft-How could the richest man in the world not be a morning person? After ensuring that he sleeps seven hours a day, he begins his day with a half an hour workout.

9.   Jack Dorsey, Co Founder, Twitter- Jack Dorsey wakes up at 5 am and follows it up with a wellness routine compromising of wellness and meditation.

10.   Julie Bowen, TV Actress- Julie Bowens fitness routines 45 minutes of running early in the morning.

11.   Richard Branson, Founder, Virgin Group- This flamboyant businessman credits his success to exercising. His routine comprises of waking up a 5 am and indulging in some kite surfing, tennis or swimming.

12.   Mark Zunckerberg, Founder, Facebook- This iconic progenitor of the social media revolution likes to exercise in the mornings too. He goes running with his dogs in the morning, three days a week.

13.   Condoleeza Rice, Former Secretary of State- Who doesn't know of Conoleeza Rice. As

secretary of state, she was equally known for her
sterling performance and her graceful demeanor.
She too is a morning exercise person, waking up
at 4:30 am to do 40 minutes of cardio on a
treadmill or eliptica machine.

14.   Tim Cook, CEO, Apple- Tim Cook not only heads
Apple, but also happens to be a morning exercise
person. His routine comprises of waking up at
4:30 am and work out in the gym. Alternatively,
he cycles and rock climbs.

15.   Ariana Huffington, Co Founder, Huffington Post-
She is not only the iconic founder of Huffingtom
Post, but also someone who takes morning
exercise seriously. She begins her day with yoga
and meditation.

16.   Jennifer Aniston, Actress- Needs no
introduction, right? Her morning workout is pretty
intense too. This incorporates a thirty minutes of a
spin yoga combination, followed by 40 minutes of
gymming. So now you know how she continues
so good after all these many years.

17.   Joanna Coles,   editor-in-chief, Cosmopolitan- Joanna Coles walks her dog at 7:30 am in the morning, including on weekends for about half an hour. This is the only time in the day that she gets entirely for herself .

18.   Gwyneth Paltrow, Actress- In spite of not being a modern person Gyneth Paltrow makes it a point to wake up at 4:30 am in the morning and perform some Yogic asnas. She ensures that she does this six days a week and when combined with eating the right kind of food, she feels right on top.

If so many of the rich and the famous, the super achievers and celebrities swear by the efficacy of a morning workout, there must be something special about it. After all, you cannot really reach the top of your game, if you aren't performing optimally at a physical and mental level.

If you took the trouble of asking these super achievers the secret behind their success they would most likely put it down to mental and physical discipline. That is why they all turn to morning exercise.

50

There is nothing that quite gives you the sharp focus and surge of energy that getting up early in the morning and indulging in an intense workout does. Anybody who dreams of making it really big in their chosen field, will need to show more commitment than their peers toward their chosen. Waking up early and exercising is every so often the first step.

Chapter 8

Start Little, Start Now

Given a chance. Most people would like to exercise, but a very large number of such people don't ever get started because they get intimidated by the imagery presented by the fitness industry-of super-fit model like people with impossibly good physiques.

If you are one of those who look at those gods and goddesses and say, "Nah, I can never be like those," take heart. The idea is not to participate in the Olympics or walk the ramp, but to be fit, energetic and happy. Now that too definitely requires hard work, but nothing that needs you to put in a Green Beret like effort.

Of course the fact that you plan to perform exercises in the morning,might faze you even more. This hits you with a lot of force when you have just about started exercising in the morning, what with sore limbs, tired muscles and a generally sleepy you make you imagine that you don't have it in you.

But you do; it's just that you don't realize it yet. Your body is capable of not more than you give it credit for, but you cannot hot those levels overnight. You have to take an incremental approach and get your body used to an increasingly intense workout.

The thing about fitness workouts, especially morning fitness workouts is that the very term "fitness workout" intimidates someone who finds even getting out of bed in the morning an ordeal. That is unfortunate, because it makes you lose perspective.

It is not as if you will be exercising right through the day to achieve that. Like I stated earlier, even fifteen minutes of exercise a day in the morning, if done the right way and with unfailing commitment is good enough to put you on the path of fitness.

Of course fifteen minutes a day is not going to turn anybody into the Rock. But it will definitely substantially enhance the physical and mental fitness, levels of the average person leading a regular kind of life. This can be a transformative beginning in the life of someone who till now was not doing much by way of regular exercise or workout.

Once somebody sees what even fifteen minutes of daily early morning exercise can achieve for them, they will likely like to commit more time to a more comprehensive early morning exercise routine. There is an old adage which says, the journey of a thousand miles begins with a single step. So it is with morning exercise. We all have it in us(most of us at any rate) to up our game and go out their and accomplish those early morning four mile runs that some people accomplish so easily.

The human body is constructed to run long distances. Human beings have managed to outrun horses in long distance races! But we can't realize our great potential overnight. It has to be a gradual process, where our body is by and by acquainted with its own potential to perform.

Your body is not an automobile, where you can rev up the engine and away she goes. You have something called a mind that takes rational distances. Your mind knows that if you push your body too hard out of the blue, you will end up harming it. On the other hand however, if you prepare your body for the long haul ahead, it will not let you down.

A short early morning workout session does not even require any fancy equipment. An alarm clock, a pair of jogging shoes and if it is not too much trouble a pair of dumbbells are all the tools and accessories that you are ever going to need.

Think of learning to perform exercises as trying to get an education. You start by enrolling in kindergarten and progress your way through various levels to arrive at the top of your game. If you don't go through the process you will not acquire the skills to carve out a career path for yourself.

So it is with exercise. You really have to start at a very basic level and then enhance your level as you go along, till you are able to withstand and benefit from a really intense daily workout routine. People who choose not to exercise do themselves-their minds and bodies a great disservice.

Your body and mind are God's gift to you which you should take care of and nurture, for everything flows from there. By not exercising, you risk atrophying your mind and body. Not only will your life span be shorter, your quality of life will be much poorer.

Where starting with a shorter period of morning exercise scores over a longer one is that it will not leave you feeling drained. Besides, it will help you understand that early morning exercise is not a daily chore, but a daily necessity just as breakfast is. Can you imagine missing breakfast three days in a row? No, because that would be bad for you. Similarly, not exercising every day in the morning is equally bad, if not worse for you.

This is scientific fact and not a canard spread by the health and fitness industry. By starting little and starting now you will not only have taken the first important steps toward total fitness, but also understood that early morning exercise is as important for you as your daily meals.

With an epidemic of obesity and lifestyle diseases, staring the nation in the face, it is high time that everyone understood that it will take very little to comprehensively reverse the trend. Most people get trapped in their unhealthy lifestyles more on account of ignorance about how easy it is for everyone to take the initiative to reclaim their own lives.

If you are one of those people who has always secretly worried out about your health and well being and want to make a change to your sedentary lifestyle, the time to act is now. Surely anyone can spare fifteen minutes in the morning to bring about the greatest transformation in one's life.

Chapter 9

You Are Who You Want To Be

Think of the person you admire the most in life. It could be anyone –a celebrity, a member of your family, a politician, a film star, just about anyone. What is it that you like about them? Their dynamism, their infectious smile, their exuding confidence, energy and vitality. How you wish you could be like them?

Who says you can't? You can be anything or anybody you want. If you decide to improve the quality of your life, that is what you will do, provided your commitment to do so is real. If your body performs at its peak your energy levels will be such that you will be able achieve the kind of growth in life that you always wanted. You will be able to live your life with such passion that you will be a source of inspiration to others.

The trouble with most people who want to become super achievers is the fact that they put their minds and bodies through an inordinate amount of strength which creates problems for them in the long run. They forget that their bodies are their biggest allies in their quest for growth and not their foes that they have to subjugate and ill-treat.

People ill treat their bodies in myriad ways. They do so by overeating, not exercising and sleeping less. Instead of helping them get closer to their life's goals unhealthy bodies slow them down and make them inefficient. To use a metaphor to explain this take the case of the armed forces of a nation.

If they don't take good care of their men and equipment, they are not going to be able to defend their nations, if a war were to break out. That is the reason why the military has always drilled and practiced in peace time. That is what we need to bring to our personal lives-the discipline to exercise every day and eat right. We will do so if we really have set ourselves some goals in life. We will do so if we want to lead a life of purpose and fulfillment.

Our biggest problem is that we take our bodies for granted. Though nature has made our bodies extremely resilient, we have to do our bit to enable our bodies to cope with the ravages of ageing, the stresses of modern living, the toxic fat laden diet of processed food and genetic susceptibility to certain kinds of diseases. The only weapons we have against this are regular exercise and a well regulated an sensible diet.

While these may be the only two weapons available to us in our fight to reclaim our health, these are extremely powerful ones. You could liken them to a nuclear arsenal that you possess in your armory. With regular exercise and a sensible diet, you can prevent the onset of a host of lifestyle diseases, improve your immunity, increase your stamina and enhance your zest for life. You can become the man or woman you always wanted to be.

Though it has been mentioned many times in this book, there is need to remind oneself of the benefits of regular exercise. Here they are, listed in greater detail for your benefit, all over again-

    1.   Lower blood pressure

2.   Higher HDL (also known as good cholesterol)

3.   Lower LDL (also known as bad cholesterol

4.   Enhanced metabolism

5.   Optimal blood sugar levels

6.   Better mood

7.   Better bone density

8.   Stronger joints

Now that we well and truly know what the basic benefits of exercise, particularly early morning exercise are; we can start looking at how much advantage we can leverage for ourselves from it. The thing about exercise is that the more seriously you take it, the more serious are the benefits that accrue from it.

You would be amazed at how much you can push yourself to achieve, when you make exercise a part of your life. Say you are someone who breaks out into a sweat at the very thought of running a few meters. You won't imagine yourself ever being able to run a marathon in a million years. Yet you can. You may not believe so, but I am telling you, you can(unless of course there are medical reasons for your not being able to do so).

But of course, you need to be very fit to withstand the rigors of a marathon. However, it is very much within the realm of the possible to get to the stage where you can be that fit. It will take six months of training though. Think that it is not possible?

Well I don't blame you, but you would be surprised at the number of people who were in the same boat as you, but now regularly run marathons. The idea behind my telling you this is not to make you run a marathon(though that would be a most laudable objective!), but to convey to you that you have it within you to literally go forth and achieve any goal that you set yourself.

Your mind is a great tool that God has equipped you with. It can wreak miracles if you allow it to. The best thing about the mind is that you can always change its disposition if you try hard enough. If you are someone who hates to read, you can change that about yourself and become a lover of books, if you train your mind to do so. The neural pathways that carry messages and commands from the brain to the rest of the body become set in a certain way if you keep thinking a certain way.

If you tell yourself, you are a couch potato, a couch potato you shall be, However, if you make a conscious effort to become a fitness freak, with time your neural pathways will start conveying that message to your body. So you see, you can be who you want to be.

Chapter 10

Advantages of Running in The Morning

The multibillion dollar fitness industry will give you all manner of advice about the best exercise routine to follow, the diet to adopt and the lifestyle to aspire to. While all very well intentioned, this surfeit of information is likely going to leave you very confused and unsure about what you really should be doing.

Well the advice that one really should be following should be to keep it simple. And what can be simpler than going for a morning run, something that people have been doing since the dawn of mankind. Man, in fact is born to run. Modern man evolved in the savanna grasslands of Africa in a manner that made long distance running a part of his basic physiology.

If it weren't for the fact that evolution made the human race primed for long distance running we wouldn't have such humongous numbers of people routinely running over forty kilometer long marathons! In the very ancient past when man was nothing more than a bunch of hunting savages, chasing down a prey was often the only way of obtaining food and surviving. This instinct is hardwired into all of us.

That is why we all feel so good after a particularly intense bit of running. It therefore follows that one really doesn't need to sign up with an expensive health club to stay fit. All that one needs to do is to run, something we are literally born to do. Why running in the morning is particularly good is the fact that it does offer a number of psychological and physical benefits.

These include, among other things lower blood pressure, reduced stress levels and above all a great feeling of wellbeing arising from the accomplishment of something positive so early in the morning. Then there is the fact that morning times are safer times from the point of view of there being fewer pollutants and less dust in the air.

Another thing about morning running is the fact that more than the great physical benefits that an early morning run provides, it is the mental and psychological benefits that are truly awesome. Here is a whole list of them-

1. Helps Overcome Depression- The act of running makes the brain trigger the release of neurotransmitters like dopamine and serotonin, which helps restore mental health. The fact that you run first thing in the morning means, that your day begins on a good note.

2. Early Morning Running Instills Confidence- Motivating yourself to go for an early morning run day after day, will make you feel better about the fact that you could do it. Then comes the challenge of increasing the distance you run every day. With every goal that you achieve, your level of self confidence goes up.

    If you do this on a daily basis, this becomes your defining trait and you begin to carry forth this confidence in your activities and dealings through the day.

3.   Early Morning Running Keeps Your Mind Young- Nothing is sadder than a mind that has degenerated with age. The best way to prevent that is to make early morning running a daily routine. What this does is to prevent something known as neurodegeneration or slowing down of the brain. Your memory and ability to keep on learning stays as sharp as ever and your quality of life continues to be as good as before.

4.   Early Morning Running Is Good For Focus- When you run early in the morning, you effectively rev yourself up for a great day ahead. This is on account of your feeling very fresh because of the extra flow of oxygen into your brain, caused by an increase in your blood circulation. Consequently, you feel all charged up to take on whatever challenges come your way during the day.

5.   Early Morning Running Is Good For Your Sleep- If you are in the habit of early morning running, you will never have trouble falling asleep. Why

early morning running is better is that it will make you less likely to miss a workout due to unscheduled events that are more likely to occur later.

Besides, if you run or exercise closer to bed time you may not be able to fall asleep on time because of the enhancement in your body's rate of metabolism. Running in the morning on the other hand will put you just in the right frame of mind to sleep, by the time it is evening.

6.   Makes You Give Up Unhealthy Cravings- You begin your day with a vigorous run of an hour or so, you are far more likely to make healthy diet choices than if you don't. Running will more likely make you choose vegetables and fruit over fried food, drugs or alcohol.

They say that the best things in life are for free. You can't put a price on the love of your family and the companionship of your friends. The same could be said of early morning running. While it costs you nothing other than the price of a pair of running shoes, what it gives to you in return is priceless.

Anybody can run, regardless of their age and sex, as long as they haven't been forbidden from doing so by the doctor. You can do so at a place you are comfortable with and by and by increasing the intensity with time. Remember regular running is the key here, more than how long or intense your run is. It is far better to run for twenty minutes every morning, than running for an hour and a half for two days and then forgetting all about it for the next two months.

The next time you feel demotivated to put on your running shoes, remember that this is something that nature expected you to do. The fact that man has made the progress he has, stems from the ability of our ancestors to run well.

Chapter 11

Advantages of Gymming in The Morning

Of all the forms of daily morning exercise, this one takes the most commitment. You have to be really serious about your wellness to become a member of a gym, buy the necessary accessories and wake up every morning and actually head to the gym and hit it. So who are those people who do it morning after morning after morning? What motivates them to do so?

About the kind of people who don't mind getting up in the morning and pumping iron, it is the kind who are serious about their fitness and understand a bit about the science behind staying fit.

1. Boosting One's Metabolism- An early morning routine at the gym jump starts one's metabolism like nothing else. Most of us earn a living sitting behind a desk, which does nothing for our body's metabolism. Gymming first thing in the morning effectively takes care of that problem. You reach office or wherever it is that you work with your metabolism all tuned up.

2. Energy- You think gymming in the morning will drain you of all energy? Not true, it will fill you with energy. This is because you will b able to trigger the release of endorphins and other feel good endorphins that will make you feel all fresh and energized.

3. Hormonal Advantage- Like I mentioned before, a major reason for early morning gymming working out so well for us is science. Early morning is the time when the level of testosterone is highest in our bodies, enabling us to exercise more efficiently. This is because testosterone helps us in amassing muscle. Anybody who is seriously looking at enhancing their fitness level would do

well to leverage this early morning hormonal advantage.

4. Less Distractions- Morning is the time when you are least likely to be distracted or have unscheduled work upend your gymming plan for the day. Gymmin first thing in the morning is therefore a schedule you are more likely to stick to than at any other time during the day.

5. Improves Focus- A vigorous early morning workout in the gym will arouse your body like nothing else. Consequently, anything that you undertake during the course of the day will be accomplished quite easily by you.

6. Eating Healthier Food- The effort you put in to wake up early and head to the gym early in the morning is going to motivate you to make better food choices as well. This is because you don't want to fritter away the gains that you have made by exercising so intensely in the morning. So you create a kind of virtuous cycle where an early morning gymming session is followed by a day of

healthy eating followed by another gymming session the next morning.

7.   Protection Against Diabetes- People why gym first thing in the morning, even prior to having breakfast gain protection against glucose intolerance and insulin resistance, the primary markers of type 2 diabetes. So not only will you improve the way you look by gymming in the morning, you will also develop resistance against lifestyle diseases.

8.   Holistic Health Benefits Obtained By Regular Exercise- Once you have made early morning gymming your default a host of health benefits will accrue to you. These include better immunity and longevity, apart from a much happier disposition.

Chapter 12

Advantages of Swimming in The Morning

Swimming is one of the best ways to revitalize your body and mind and early morning swimming is especially so. This is on account of a number of reasons.

1.   Makes A Good Beginning To Your Day- Nothing in this world can be as refreshing as an early morning swim. For one the water is cooler at that time of the day and completely wakes you up. If you live in a warm region, an early morning swim is sure to make you feel fresh and energetic. Besides, it will help enhance your focus, setting you up for a day of productive work.

2.   Boosts Your Metabolism- An early morning swim provides a substantial boost to your metabolism, which means that your body will continue to burn calories through the course of the day.

3.	You Are More Likely To Swim In The Morning-
You are more likely to be motivated to expend the energy
required to swim early in the morning than during any
other time of the day. There is therefore less chance of
your missing your daily morning workout.

4.	A Great Way To Obtain Vitamin D- Mornings are
the time when the sun is at its mellowest and actually
helps you obtain the all important vitamin D. This is not
possible within the closed confines of an indoor gym.
Swimming in the morning therefore is the thing to do for
one more healthy reason.

5.	A Great Bouquet Of Health Benefits- Swimming
early in the morning provides one with a host of
important health benefits. It builds up your heart strength
without our having to indulge in heavy impact exercising.
That apart, it enhances your endurance, increases your
muscle strength and improves your cardiovascular fitness.
Swimming is particularly good for you in that nearly all
of our muscles are involved in a round of swimming.
Nothing like swimming to give you a full body workout
early in the morning.

6.	A Relaxing Workout- There won't be a more peaceful and relaxing workout than an early morning swim. That apart, it is a great stress buster and helps improve one's body posture and balance, while improving coordination of the limbs. The fact that it is low impact, makes it possible for those with injuries to manage to obtain a workout without aggravating their condition.

7.	Adds Variety To Your Workout- You can find a variety of places to swim-pool, river, lake or sea. The only thing to ensure is that the environment be safe for swimming. No other form of morning workout, not even running or cycling provides you with this kind of variety.

Chapter 13

Advantages Of Cycling In The Morning

Even if you are the kind of person who simply detests the very thought of exercising in the mornings, the chances are that you might not mind taking up early morning cycling. Don't believe me? Take the trouble of getting up early one morning and try your hand, or shall we say feet at cycling. You might just experience the epiphany, that you thought wasn't possible for you.

The beauty of riding a bike, very early in the morning when the sun has either made an appearance or is about to, is a little difficult to describe in words. It has to be experienced. You feel that you are the sole person on planet earth, in complete peace with yourself and in communion with nature.

Though you might be alone with only the sound of your pedalling and the tires moving on the surface of the road accompanying you, all that you feel is a sense of peace and serenity-a gratefulness for being alive. Besides, if you cycle in the mornings, even for two to four hours every week you will derive a host of benefits.

- A comprehensive workout for your muscles as it puts to use all the major muscle groups. What's more, being a low impact exercise, it does not put any inordinate stress on the body.

- Cycling does not require any complex skill, other than learning to ride. Once you have mastered that, you will never ever forget how to ride a cycle. This means that a cycle is all the equipment you will ever need to comprehensive early morning workout.

- Cycling is fun and doesn't really seem like exercise. In fact, it allows one to commune with nature as you can ride in interesting outdoor terrain of myriad types.

- The intensity of your cycling workout can easily be adjusted-from very gentle to intense. So even if you are recovering from an illness or injury you can slowly enhance the tempo of your workout.

- Cycling is a proven way of improving your strength and stamina. The more you cycle, the more your aerobic fitness improves and the stronger and fitter you become.

- Cycling can be a great way of commuting. It is not only cheaper, but far healthier also. With environmental degradation becoming a huge problem worldwide, commuting to work by cycle.

- Cycling is particularly good at improving joint mobility. So if you want to keep those joints in fine shape, all you need to do is pedal away every morning.

- Cycling is a great stress buster. Beginning your day with a round of cycling will not only rid your body of any overnight stress, but also leave you fresh and invigorated for the rest of the day.

- There is nothing like cycling to improve your posture and improve the coordination of your limbs. If the stresses and rigors of daily life have negatively impacted the way you carry yourself , taking to cycling early in the morning will help you restore your posture and improve limb coordination.

- We tend to lose bone strength as we grow older. What cycling does is help strengthen our bones and withstand ageing better.

- If you make it a point to cycle every morning you will be able to bring down your body fat levels. This in turn results in a host of health benefits including lower susceptibility to heart disease and diabetes.

- Cycling is quite effective in chasing away your blues. People who cycle everyday in the morning report significantly lower levels of anxiety and depression.

- Obesity, which is another name for a chronic weight problem and has assumed the proportions of an epidemic can be tackled quite effectively with early morning exercising. By cycling you can burn as much as 300 calories an hour. Even half an hour of cycling will burn as much as 5 kilograms of fat in a year.

- Cycling even helps reduce the chances of bowel cancer.

- Cycling, especially, helps people with osteoarthritis because it is a low intensity exercise.

- Because cycling helps reduce stress and anxiety, it is a great way of warding off mental illness

Making it a habit to cycle regularly in the mornings helps you be in the pink of your mental and physical health. What's more of all the workouts, this is the least bothersome and the most enjoyable one. The best thing is that it does not require any training and supervision and all that one needs is the ability to ride a cycle.

One can take to early morning cycling, to enjoy the bounties of nature in the shape of fresh air, a gentle sun and a spectacular vista if one is cycling by the sea or in the mountains. One might even cycle to work and combine an environment friendly commute with a morning workout.

Chapter 14

Morning Exercises to Lose Fat Around The Belly

While all extra fat around the body is bad, belly fat is the worst. This is as true aesthetically, as it is medically. A pot belly apart from making a person look fat and ungainly is an indication of poor health and makes one susceptible to a host of diseases ranging from cholesterol and heart ailments to strokes and diabetes.

This is the reason why a reduction of belly fat is one of the focus areas of any regular exercise or workout regime. Here again, mornings are a particularly advantageous time to perform exercises that help reduce belly fat. However, this is something that needs to be approached scientifically and not in an unplanned or haphazard manner.

Like you can't just have a go at crunches or sit-ups because you feel that you are directly targeting the belly area and will consequently lose fat there. Neither can you be aimlessly indulging in aerobic exercise hoping to knock down the belly fat by burning calories.

Among the most effective morning exercise that will help you shed those unwanted pounds around your belly are resistance exercises. This helps you create the lean muscle tissue that will help you shed belly fat. Any work our that helps you build lean muscle tissue will kick-start your metabolism in ways that will make you continue to burn calories through the day.

What also helps with removing stubborn belly fat is something called high intensity interval training. This involves your alternating between fast paced, intense bursts of cardio exercise with standing core exercises. The things to do with trying to reduce belly fat is use targeted strategy, rather than continuing to exercise in a certain way, hoping that the belly fat will go away.

The reason why mornings are a good time to try and reduce belly fat is the fact that mornings are a great time for trying out different variations of technique; something that is a must in one's attempt to lose belly fat. You are far more likely to follow a short but intense workout regimen early morning,in the comfort of your home, than you are going to be able to accomplish it in a couple of hour workout in an expensive gym.

The mere expedient of performing an intense and brief early morning workout followed by a nutritious breakfast is going to make you three to four times more likely to both make healthier decisions, including eating ones during the rest of the day. This could actually result in your losing between four to ten pounds in a month's time. You continue doing this for another four to six months and you would have tranformed yourself as well as your lifestyle. You will lose the extra weight that you had been carrying all along and very importantly you would lose it around your belly.

The amazing thing is that you can spend as little as eight to fifteen minutes performing these intense circuit workouts and obtain genuine weight loss including from around the belly. Losing belly fat has a multitude of benefits. The most important of course is the fact that you get to improve your longevity and reduce the chances of premature death. That apart you look your best, which greatly enhances your self esteem and is therefore very good for your mental well being. That apart you feel more energized, on account of your much enhanced metabolism and area able to perform at your productive best at whatever you undertake.

I stated earlier that resistance exercises are more effective in helping one lose belly fat than cardio exercises and that is largest true. However, cardio exercises do play a part in our battle against the belly bulge and cannot be given the go by. A 15 to 20 minute walk in the morning on an empty stomach does help in burning fat. But it has to be complimented by strength training involving abdominal and core toning exercises. This includes exercises like crunches, planks and v sits.

Now that you know what is required for you to attack that stubborn belly fat- a combination of resistance and cardio performed intensely, you have got to keep at it consistently, every morning. The problem with losing belly fat is that it requires one to be steadfast in one's efforts. Easy as it is to acquire belly fat losing it is quite difficult.

Quite often people give up their efforts to get their belly in shape because of the seeming lack of progress. Well, the thing is that you have to accept that you will have to work hard to get rid of that excess fat at the wrong place. The best way to speeden the process is to eat the right kind of food alongside peforming the right kind of exercises.

You have to learn to give up all kinds of processed and high fat food. That means no more steaks, pizzas, burgers, colas and alcohol. You should go easy in sugar and salt as well. Eating fresh fruits, vegetables, nuts and pulses in place of the above will help as well

What you really require to do, is to make a comprehensive lifestyle change with starts with exercising first thing in the morning. A pot belly is a sure indicator of a lifestlye gone awry. The best way to deal with it is to change the way you live your days starting from the moment you get up.

You don't have to dedicate a huge amount of time to your morning workouts, as I explained above. What you need instead is dedication, consistency and the right technique. Combine that with a sensible diet and you will see the last of your belly fat.

Chapter 15

Morning Exercise Tales

Hardly anyone takes to morning exercise naturally. Who wants to leave the comfort of bed and put oneself through a punishing schedule. However, there are hordes of people who come to love the routine of waking up early in the morning and exercising vigorously. They love the fact that it makes them fit to take on the rigors of the day ahead. The fact that they don't have to head to a gym after a day spent working adds to the charm of a morning workout. They can now use their freed up time with family and friends and be happier individuals on account of that.

There certainly is something mystical about waking up early and heading out to exercise, especially if you do it outdoors. Perhaps it has something to do with our caveman past when our ancestors lived lives that were far more in sync with nature and the elements. For every extra hour you spend in bed you lose out on fifteen days in a year. That may not seem much, but remember we are not here forever. Every minute of our life that gets spent is never going to come back.

Waking up in the morning frees up more time for us to cherish life. Perhaps that is why early mornings often give us a spiritual vibe. The ancient Indians would wake up early in the morning and offer salutations to the morning sun by way of performing a series of yogi exercises known as suryanamaskar.

Not only do the early morning suryanamaskar exercises cause you to have good physical health, but put you in a good mental state. This is because, apart from the performing physical exercise you are also expressing gratitude to the sun for sustaining life on earth. Science tells you that expressing gratitude has a positive bearing upon our mental health, leading us to lead much happier and healthier lives.

A lot of the positivity that surrounds morning exercise is in the mental realm. The physical and the mental are in fact dependent upon each other. A good mental state promotes a good physical state and vice versa. There are a number of reasons fir morning exercises being great for mental health-

Helps Overcome Depression- A number of studies have shown that exercise has the ablity to treat minor depression as well as antidepressant. Anybody who suffers from minor expression would likely get rid of it if they exercised first thing in the morning. This would help the body release feel-good endorphins, which would mark a happy beginning to that person's day.

If that person does this on a regular basis, his or her neural patterns would become healthier, making them a much happier and sorted kind of individual. Besides, early morning exercise helps disrupt a negative thought pattern that would trap one in depression

Helps Alleviate Anxierty- People who exercise first thing in the morning are less likely to experience anxiety than the ones who do not. This is because early morning workouts relieve stress and tension, besides boosting one's physical and mental faculties. This helps you view things in the right perspective, thereby making you less prone to any kind of anxiety.

Helps Overcome ADHD- Early morning exercise is an effective way of handling Attention Deficit Hyperactivity Syndrome on account of its ability to help one enhance one's concentration, memory, focus and mood. This is because physical activity is known to give a boost to a brain's ability to increase dopamine, serotonin, and norepinephrine levels in the body, all of which have a bearing on focus and attention.

Helps Deal With Symptoms of PTSD- Early morning exercise helps one deal with the symptoms of post traumatic stress disorder, on account of its ability to overcome stress and anxiety. By focusing on the process of exercise one can block out the negative thoughts one was obsessing about. Exercises involving the movement of both arms and legs are the ones that are the most helpful ones-swimming, running, weight training, rock climbing, whitewater rafting and so on.

Better Memory And Thinking Ability- The fact that when you exercise early in the morning you trigger the release of endorphins, means that you are in a better mental shape to take on tasks and accomplish them. Besides, exercise helps stimulate the creation of new brain cells thereby delaying ageing.

Early Morning Exercise Helps Enhance Self Esteem- If you are able to get up early day after day after day, come what may you would have shown the ability to exercise tremendous self discipline and will power. This will not only help you to improve your health, but also give you a feeling of achievement that will boost your self esteem.

Resilience- People who are able to muster the will to exercise early every morning are likely to be more resilient than the ones who are not. They are likely to be tougher physically and mentally and will be able to take the challenges of life head-on. There is very little likelihood of such people turning to drugs or alcohol when faced with a crisis situation.

The thing about morning exercises is that you don't have to be intimidated at the thought of performing them. As explained many times earlier in the book, you don't even have to spend a very long time working out. You can even begin with eight to fifteen minute long workout routines. What is important is that you should do it. You can increase the intensity and duration by and by as you begin to notice the benefits.

Chapter 16

Why it is Important to Promote Morning Exercise

There is an obesity epidemic facing the US. Nearly 40% of the adults and about 20% of the adults are obese. On the whole a catastrophically high figure of more than 70% of the American population fall either under the overweight or obese category. Shockingly Americans with a normal BMI of less than 25 are now in a minority.

What is worrisome is the apparent lack of will among vast sections of obese and fat people to do anything about losing weight. To that add the fact that people consume huge amounts of processed food and don't seem to exercise enough and you have a really worrisome situation at hand. The obesity epidemic is leading to conditions of blood pressure, diabetese, stroke and heart diseases leading to millions of avoidable deaths every year.

The cost of obesity related medical bills is a humongous $190 billion every year. Then there are the many man-hours lost on account of illness causing a loss to the national economy. The only thing that can reverse this trend is an overhauling of people's lifestyles.

People have to be made to understand the grave risk that obesity causes them. This has to be conveyed to them by the government, media, social organizations and other advocacy groups. They have to be told that just because there is easy availability of processed and refined food it does not mean that they can't make healthy food choices.

Similarly they have to be made aware of the necessity of leading an active lifestyle. Not that everyone has to train for a marathon (though that wouldn't be a bad idea as well). What they do need to do is to consider incorporating regular exercise albeit on a minor scale to start with. The best way for them to embark upon that path is by adopting the path of daily morning exercise.

The best way to make something an intrinsic part of your daily routine is by doing it the first thing in the morning-like brushing your teeth and having your breakfast. If you come to understand that early morning workouts, whatever they might be and howsoever long or short, are essential for a good quality of life, you will make it a part of your life.

The biggest advantage of opting for early morning workouts is the fact that one is more likely to stay the course than if one scheduled it later in the day. Working out early makes a person fresh and energetic through the day. If you schedule it toward the evening you may often not be able to undertake your workout due to fatigue or being overtaken by the events of the day. Besides, you may prioritize pending time with the family over exercise.

The most disciplined of all types of organizations are the armed forces. Have you noticed how early morning drills are an integral part of their life. This is because the instructors know that that is the best way for recruits from diverse backgrounds to adopt a life of discipline that requires one to face many formidable physical mental challenges on am almost daily basis. The rest of their training, including classroom training happens later on in the day, because the instructors know that the rigors of the early morning drill would have primed the trainees to give their best during the rest of the day.

Working out in the morning comes with inherent advantages that include a more efficient workout resulting in better physical and mental conditioning of the people undergoing it. If people were motivated on a national basis to give early morning workouts a shot, a large proportion of them would likely make it a long term habit.

As the benefits of early morning workouts would start accruing over a length of time, they would start increasing the amount of time invested by them in their workouts resulting in even better results. This would encourage them to advocate early morning exercise to their peers, who would then do their bit advocating the cause.

To use the terminology of the digital age, the task of advocating early morning exercise should be carried out on a viral basis. There has to be a buzz around the concept. People have to be made to understand that early morning exercise should be considered as critically important as getting vaccinated against diseases. As a matter of fact that is exactly what early morning workouts help you achieve-protection against a host of deadly diseases like heart diseases, diabetes, stroke and blood pressure.

Apart from these lifestyle diseases, early morning exercises also help ward off diseases pertaining to the degeneration of the brain because of Alzheimer's. Presently there is no known cure for Alzheimer's and prevention is the best way to deal with it. Alzheimer's not only devastates the lives of millions of elderly relatives, but also causes immense grief to their loved ones.

If we could motivate more and more Americans to take to early morning exercising, we would put them on the path to not only having healthy hearts, but healthy brains as well. This means that not only will they protect their hearts against disease, but their brains as well. The simple expedient of taking some time out for an early- morning workout would both provide them with longevity as well as a better quality of life.

The easy availability of food , shelter and other comforts of life to modern man has wreaked havoc with his physiology. For ten and thousands of years man has had to hunt, scour, run and fight to be able to eat and survive. This naturally meant that mankind was used to a very vigorous lifestyle for most of its existence. Now along comes modern times and all the trouble a modern man has to take to get food is to walk up to his or her refrigerator.

So naturally mankind is unwell and upset mentally. The only way for him or her to restore balance is to eat less of the mass produced processed food and be far more active physically. He or she may still get the food from the refrigerator, but only after running for at least half an hour.   While man no longer needs to hunt for his breakfast, there is no harm in running around a park for some time simulating what his ancestor would have done tens of thousands of years ago.

It is a little ironic that as the inequality of income amongst nations gets reduced, lifestyle diseases start making an appearance across nations of the world. It is funny that in parts of the world where people survived by subsistence farming, the coming of industry would introduce processed ready made food to former subsistence peasants now working as factory workers. This would sooner than later result in their suffering from the same lifestyle diseases that people in the industrialized west suffer from.

The solution again to this problem is not to roll back the clock, but to take measures like eating a balanced diet and undertaking morning exercise. That is the best way to achieve the right balance. The very paradigm of progress has to be redefined and people need to be weaned away from dependence upon so called modern means of convenience. These include eating processed food loaded with fat, refined sugar and a high percentage of fat and using mechanized transport for even buying groceries.

Eating wholesome food comprising of cereals, fresh fruits and vegetables, nuts, and healthy oil is one part of the solution. The other part is doing more about walking and cycling rather than traveling by one's personal. One could use public transport for one's daily commute.

The best way to usher in this health revolution is to condition children in school to make morning exercise and healthy eating a part of their everyday life. Let them not get trapped in the late twentieth century hedonistic lifestyle of living to consume like there were no tomorrow. This has almost brought the planet to the brink.

The way of the twentieth century is the regenerative and holistic way. This encompasses everything about our lives. The way we eat, the way we commute, what sort of buildings we live in, what sort of fuel we use, how we dispose our waste and every other important aspect of our life. We humans need to move from our infantile fascination with what we consider progress and development and understand things in their real perspective.

The purpose of life is not to accumulate objects, at the cost of one's health and happiness, but to be happy and contented at all costs. Things like exercising early in the morning, put you firmly on that path. To that extent exercising early in the morning is amongst the most important things that you need to do. It's not some health-fad which is the flavor of the moment.

There are any number of studies that will tell you that waking up early gives you a great start in whatever you are undertaking. Students who wake up early score better in examinations than the ones who don't.

Waking up early inevitable leads you to having a better diet that is balanced and nourishing. There's no chance of someone who wakes up early to be skipping breakfast every no and then as late risers often do.

Waking up early leads to better productivity because you have a chance to plan out your day better. Above all waking up early positively impacts your mental health. How your first few hours of the morning pan out decides the fate of the rest of the day. People who are habituated to waking up early are usually the disciplined sort who are able to plan the rest of the day with clarity of thought and focus. If people make a conscious effort to become early risers they will be able become mentally stronger leading to a host of concomitant benefits.

Morning people are invariably happy people. If you add daily exercise to your morning routine you will turbo charge the goodness that accrues from becoming an early morning person. Your physical and mental health will improve manifold and your life will take on a different hue-of super success, super achievement and super contentment.

Chapter 17

Morning Mental Exercises

Almost all of the morning exercises that have been described in this book have been physical exercises, though they have always had a bearing on a person's mental well-being as well. That being stated there are morning exercises that are more mental in nature than physical. However, here again the beneficial impact of these exercises are both mental and physical. You never really can't separate the mental from the physical, when it comes to human beings.

1. Listening To Music- Listening to gentle classical music in the morning has a beneficial impact on the human brain. There have been a number of studies that have liked listening to music to a number of long term positive impacts-like enhancement of a person's special temporal

reasoning, increase in work output, improvement in verbal fluency, better cognitive functioning and so on.

Listening to music early in the morning is a great way to be happy, positive, calm and happy. This will naturally translate into better physical health as well.

2. Keeping A Gratitude Journal- Now you might wonder what kind of an early morning exercise is that- a most effective one kept by a whole lot of extremely successful men and women from around the world. The reason for this is that it allows one to see things in the right perspective. Instead of cribbing about what you don't have, you started showing appreciation for what you did have your mental and physical health would improve.

More than your material possession it is the gift of life you should be grateful for. You should be grateful for the love of your family, the support of your friends, the bounties of nature like food and sunshine. You are not going to live forever and everything you take for granted today, will not exist tomorrow.

So find the time every morning to write down about five things that you will be grateful for that day. In just three weeks of doing so you will find yourself to be a significantly happier person.

3. Meditation- This is one early morning exercise that has been around for thousands of years. Science has validated a host of benefits that accrue on account of this early morning mental exercise. Meditation can help us improve focus, reduce anxiety, relieve us of depression and improve our overall mental makeup.

    People who meditate regularly every morning have a much improved ability to remember things much more efficiently than the ones who don't on account of their ability to blank out what's irrelevant. This gives one the ability to perform better in whatever they take up.

4. Play A Logic Based Game- Playing a logic based game in the morning can help rev up your brain. Games like crossword puzzles, scrabble, quizzes

improves cognitive abilities. This is especially beneficial to those who are getting along in years. Theses days one can even download games that help tone our mental muscles and keep diseases like dementia, Alzheimer's at bay. As with physical exercises, these mental exercises need to be done regularly for them to be fully effective.

5. Reading The Newspaper- Reading the newspaper in the morning has been a tradition in most families ever since the advent of daily newspapers. Though people are increasingly reading news via the Internet, this is one habit from the old days, they would do well to preserve. Early morning newspaper reading keeps you up to date with the goings on around the world, as well helps keep your mind sharp.

6. Doing A Recall Exercise- This exercise begins with your creating a list. Any kind of list-say things to do this week. Now memorize the contents of the list and hide it away. Try recall the list after an hour and see how many items you can remember without referring to the list. Morning is

a good time to perform this mental exercise, both because you are at your freshest and more likely to have the time.

7.   Doing Mental Calculations- The dependence upon electronic calculating devices has not done our minds any great favors. Try doing calculations totally mentally, not even using pen and paper and see how you fare. Again, you will find mornings a very conducive time for his kind of an activity.

8.   Drawing A Map From Memory- If you go for early morning jogs or cycling head out in a different direction every day. After you come back home tray and draw a map from your memory and see how you fare.

9.   Have A Variety Of Different Breakfast- Challenging your myriad senses is a great way of exercising your brain. If the smell of bacon and eggs is the smell you associate with breakfast, try and shape up things a bit. Start having fruits for breakfast for some time and let the smell of apples and peaches define breakfast for you now!

10. Try Using your Other Hand- If you are used to writing with your right hand try writing with the left hand instead. Mornings are a good time to carry out this little experiment. Other things you can try doing in the mornings with your weaker hand could be brushing your teeth. This switching of hands is known to be a great brain exercise that keeps your mind very active and agile and better able to withstand aging.

The difficulty you will experience in doing this at first is precisely what is going to benefit your brain. So keep at it.

11. Take Your Morning Shower With Your Eyes Closed- This is a great way of making your brain create new neural pathways, as it will have to figure out new ways of managing a familiar routine. Instead of vision you will have to use the sense of touch to figure out things.

12. Take A New And Unfamiliar Route To Your Office Every Morning- This is a great way to activate the cortex and hippocampus areas of your

brain. Sticking to the same old routine on the other hand does nothing to stimulate the brain.

I mentioned earlier that it is not necessary that only mental exercises be the ones that your directly stimulate the mind. Even physical exercises help in doing that by helping create new neural connections. This helps one improve memory and keep the aging of the brain in check. Then again physical exercise increases the flow of oxygen rich blood to the brain and fortifying it with glucose while carrying away the waste. What better time to augment that fresh supply of oxygen than early morning.

Besides, it helps to enhance the growth of cerebral blood vessels. At the same time physical exercise also helps provide stimulation to the brain's synapses because of its ability to preserve the many acetylcholine receptors found at the point where muscles and nerves meet. Active people like the ones who exercise in the morning have more of these receptors in their brains than the ones who don't. Physical exercise is actually as much brain food as mental exercise is. The thing is that even a moderate amount of exercising that can easily be accomplished in the mornings is good for the brain.

Its All About The Brain Cells- A study undertaken by the Salk Instituute in 1999 showed for the first time that unlike what was previously thought adults can grow new brain cells by a process known as neurogenesis. Physical exercise is the catalyst that enables this fascinating regeneration known as neurogenesis. How it does is by producing a brian protein known as Noggin, which is responsible for both neurogenesis and the creation of stem cells. Running is particularly suited to aid this process and if you could make a daily morning run an indispensible part of your life, you can be pretty certain that your brain will continue to be in top shape right up to a very old age.

What this study brought to the fore is nothing short of revolutionary and it is important that we realize that we can actually enhance our level of intelligence.

- Intelligence is not finite and can be enhanced with the help of the right stimulus. This means we can always get better and do better. It doesn't matter what we were endowed with at birth.

- The more we exercise and train our brain the better it gets to be.

- You have it within yourself to enhance our cognitive abilities, irrespective of what stage you are at. This means that you can essentially be what you want to be, if you try hard enough.

- The act of cognitive enhancement in one area can augment abilities in totally unrelated areas.

Chapter 18

Becoming A Morning Person

By now you would well and truly have understood that exercising in the morning is wonderful and results in a host of benefits accruing to us that substantially enhance our quality of life. So what's there to not like about early morning exercise, right? But therein lies the problem. Most people or at any rate many people are not morning people. Morning is when they are at their grumpiest and the least inclined to indulge in any kind of exercise-mental or physical.

But the fact of the matter is that if one is desirous of achieving something major in life they cannot do so without iron-clad discipline. Getting up early in the morning, full of beans and enthusiasm, is one of the outcomes of that kind of discipline. Morning people come with a huge advantage over everybody else in that they do things first by getting up earlier than they really have to.

For them the time before work is a sacred time. This is the time in which they focus on what matters to them. In doing so, they often achieve by breakfast what others often don't do in a day's work. How do they do it, morning after morning? Can everybody do it, or is it a special kind of person who is naturally endowed with this life transforming ability of being able to wake up fresh as a daisy morning after morning after morning?

Of course you can do it. You just need to get your schedule right. The reason that many people feel that there is something wrong with them and they are not morning people is that they mess up their schedules. If you are going to be spending time watching TV till late in the night every day, you are naturally not going to want to wake up early the next morning. The very simple expedient of going to bed early is going to ensure that you will wake up earlier and fresher the next morning.

But this is not really rocket science and you know it already. True, but what is obvious, needs to be pointed out sometimes. All the same, getting up early day after day after day is easier said than done. You know you have tried several times, but inevitably relapsed into your old unhealthy routine. But there are steps that you can take to make it possible for you to become a morning person after all. Here's what you can do-

- Maintain A Consistent Sleep Schedule- You can't be erratic with you sleep schedule-sleeping early and then alternately sleeping late and expect to be able to become a morning person. If you realize that you need to start sleeping early, please do that gradually, fifteen minutes at a time. Once you have managed to start sleeping at the ideal time, you will hit a sweet stop and wake up fresh and enthusiastic every morning.

- Maintain The Right Work-Life Balance-Often, it is just a case of maintaining the right work-life balance. If you are working late every night even to the extent of harming your health, you are not being very wise, for sooner or later your body and mind will buckle under the strain. You can hardly expect to become a morning person in such circumstances.

Getting your work-life balance right is one of the prerequisites of trying to prepare yourself to become a morning person. This will require or you to by and by do away with your evening commitments and appointments, so that you are able to retire to bed at a sensible hour so as to wake up refreshed the next morning.

- Take Naps- It is quite possible, perhaps inevitable that in spite of your best efforts, you end up having a sleep deficit. Try and take naps whenever you can to make up your lost sleep. Churchill did that right through the Second World War!

- Remove Screens From The Bedroom- Do you end up watching TV before sleeping every night? Banish the TV from your bedroom. Do you carry your phone and laptop to bed? Don't do that. On second thoughts, keep the phone and set up an alarm for the next morning.

Your bedroom should be a place where you retire to relax and sleep, not work or entertain. Try not to watch any television and hour before going to bed.

  - If You Are Tired Sleep- You may have a certain designated time for sleeping but if one some occasion your body is telling you that you should sleep, then that is what you should be doing. Don't force your mind to think that it is okay to press on with work, when you are clearly quite tired.

  - Leave your bedroom as soon as you are up- You did very well to make your bedroom very conducive to relaxing and sleeping. But it is not right to linger in that environment, once you are up. You might want to walk to the kitchen and get a glass of water to get completely out of sleep mode.

- Wake Up The Same Time Every Morning-Choose an early morning time that you would like to wake up and stick to that. This will make your body habituated to that time and your internal body clock will ensure that you wake up at that time day after day after day.

- Make Provision For Natural Light-Haven't you noticed how you energized the moment you move out in sunlight. Sit by a window when you make up to catch a glimpse of the sun and feel a surge of energy pass through you. If you live in a cold place where winters are general dark and gray, try installing a sun lamp to make your body clock operate normally.

- Have Something To Look Forward To The Next Day- Do you remember the time in school when you couldn't wait to got to bed, so that you could get up the next morning and head for the school picnic? Having something to look forward to the next day puts you in a good mood and you are up in a jiffy he next morning, because you have something to look forward to.

It might be a school friend you are seeing, going to watch a game of basketball or even catching a movie. Looking forward to the coming day with anticipation will make you get up early alright.

- Have A Hearty Breakfast- Let's face it. Getting up early in the morning is tough on you. The least you can do is to make things a little easy by having a hearty breakfast. A night of sleeping lowers our blood sugar levels and rate of metabolism. It is important that we fortify ourselves with a great breakfast-think proteins, veggies and whole-grain.

- Give Yourself A Reward- Waking up early requires discipline and dedication. However, one can think of rewarding oneself by showing the will and discipline to make it possible. Use the extra time you get by waking up early by doing something you like, for instance reading a fashion magazine or a blog by your favorite blogger.

- Remember It Is Beautiful In The Morning- You have got to remember what it is like getting up early in the morning, becoming a morning person. Just imagine yourself watching the sun rising over the horizon. If you live in a valley, you know how spectacular the sight of the sun peeping over the mountains looks. Those who live in a place that has the sea on their east know just how glorious a sunrise by the sea looks.

No photograph or painting can match the brilliant hues that nature paints. Morning time is the time to commune with nature. The best thing is that you can do this almost every single day of your life, if that is what you want to do. Early mornings take you away from the cacophony of daily life-television blaring, traffic drowning out every other sound, children screaming their lungs out, your neighbors playing music at the loudest and so on.

Instead, you hear bird-song, the leaves rustling in the breeze, the air smelling of morning dew and foliage. Maybe you will feel like saying a prayer, even if you are not a believer.

- Create The Right Mindset- The number of hours available to people are the same everywhere. Yet there are some who seem to have more than it than the others. How's that possible? You have got to train the mind to view the time available to you and how it can be best utilized in a very different way from what you have been doing.

It's all about optimal usage of time. That necessarily has to include how you feel during different times of the day. Mornings are the time when you feel at your freshest (hopefully). As the day progresses, your involvement in your daily activities increases, while you efficiency reduces in direct proportion. As the evening approaches, you feel more and more tired, but you press on regardless.

By the time you fall asleep, it is late in the night, and you do not wake up at your freshest the next morning. You have got to learn to manage your time better. That means that you should have great starts to your mornings. This should extend through the day enabling you to work with optimal efficiency, so that you have no need to work late. This would create a virtuous cycle of your sleeping on time and waking up early fresh and raring to go.

You can do it, if you change your mindset from can't do it to can do it.Once you find that it is no longer a problem waking up early in the morning, you can have it all. Great health, great career and great personal life. You will find it quite easy to take the right decisions like exercising, eating the right kind of food and keeping away from stressful situations.

Chapter 19

Exercising In The Mornings

This book has dealt with the advantages of exercising in the mornings at considerable length. However, it is possible that in the large amount of information that one has shared about the dynamics of exercising in the mornings, one may lose sight of the core message- You have got to exercise in the morning.

So the last chapter of the book will in a sense summarize and paraphrase what the rest of the book says. The principal reason for wanting to understand the dynamics of exercising in the mornings is the fact that it apparently has a paradigm changing impact on the way we live life. It makes super-achievers out of people who seem to have fallen into a rut with no hope of redeeming themselves or achieving their most cherished aspirations.

Waking up in the morning and working out, if done on a regular basis transforms your life. One there is less likelihood of your missing a workout due to the events of the day overtaking you. Two you get more work accomplished. Three your day gets filled with positivity and physical vitality, allowing you to work better. Four you are able to achieve better work-life balance. Lastly, it is great for physical and mental health.

Specifically, it helps in the following ways:

1. Improves Metabolism- The human body burns more calories after a workout. So if you have a workout the first thing in the morning, the benefits accrue through the day, even though you may be only sitting behind your work desk punching away at the computer keyboard.

    This happens on account of Excess Post Exercise Oxygen Consumption(EPOC). According to one study, people who have worked out in the morning burn an extra 190 calories in the fourteen hours that follow, when compared with those who did not exercise.

2.   Enhances Physical And Mental Energy- Nothing wakes up the mind and preps the body better than early morning exercising. You feel physically energized post an early morning workout, while your focus and mental ability get sharpened as well. All in all, you get primed to perform.

It has been found out that post exercise cognitive improvement at 12% is higher than the 6% obtained by drinking coffee.

3.   Improves Self Discipline- You will only wake up early every day to workout id you are able to muster the will and determination to do so. That you can, signifies the fact that you have been able to improve self discipline. The good news though is that the longer you are able to stay the course, the easier it is for you to exercise discipline.

Another positive spin off of developing the discipline to get up early every day to exercise is the fact that it spills over to other aspects of your life. For e instance, you may take to eating sensibly since you don't want to fritter away the gains of your workout.

4.   Helps You Obtain Your Fitness Goals- The very raison d'etre of of early morning exercising is fitness. If you are going to take the trouble of waking up early every morning and indulging in a vigorous workout you are likely to ensure that you succeed in your objectives. When you do this over the long term you get into the goal oriented mind-space that can only augur well for you.

5.   Helps You Sleep Better- You make the effort to get up early every morning, you sure will be able to sleep well. This is on account of your body getting quite tired by the end of the day, prompting you to sleep with ease. The best thing about morning exercise is the fact that it improves both the duration and the quality of your sleep.

6.   Helps You Live A Better Life- People who exercise early in the morning on a regular basis, invariably live better lives. This is account on of achieving better physical and mental health. You are able to perform better at work, have wholesome personal relations and even have time for leisure in the evenings.

Besides early morning exercise is touted as a panacea for a number of ailments from colds and indigestion to depression and listlessness.

7. Wards Off Aging- People who are in the habit of exercising every morning are able to ward off aging because physical exercise actually helps regenerate brain cells. This is true of anybody irrespective of what the condition of their mental prowess and faculties might be at the tome of beginning the process of early morning exercising. This is wonderful news for those who are getting along in years and fear diminishing mental faculties. Millions of senior Americans suffer from Alzheimer's disease, a most unfortunate disease of the mind that renders one's brain progressively inefficient.

8. Warding Off Lifestyle Diseases- Lifestyle diseases like diabetes, blood pressure, stroke and heart disease can be kept at bay if one maintains a routine of exercising in the mornings. Considering that America and indeed many other parts of the world suffer from an obesity

epidemic, adopting early morning exercising can provide a way out of this humongous problem

It therefore makes sense for the government, healthcare services, schools, colleges and voluntary organizations to do their very best to advocate morning exercise for everyone. Let people understand that exercising in the mornings is as important as brushing one's teeth.

While most would agree that exercising in the morning is good for them, not everyone would be able to make the effort required. There are quite a few people who are just not morning people and cannot imagine that they could ever be that. But they can, if they follow the steps given below-

1. Built anticipation around the nest day- If you have something to look forward to the next day, like meeting an old friend, watching a movie, going on a date etc., you will wake up with enthusiasm. It likely won't take much to motivate you to work out in the morning if you are in a happy state of mind like that.

2.	Remember that even short workouts help- You don't have to get demotivated at the thought of spending a couple of hours every morning working out. Even short workouts lasting no longer than eight to fifteen minutes will benefit you. You can of course increase the duration once you begin to notice the benefits of the workout you are already performing every morning.

3.	Choose a fun workout- You don't have to sweat at the thought of sweating it out in gym every morning. You can choose the workout that suits you. There are so many options that you might actually look forward or even walking will do just as fine.

4.	Have an exercise partner join you- If you exercise along with an exercise partner, you will find it easier to develop the motivation to keep going. The two of you can both monitor each other's progress as well as encourage one another. A little bit of friendly competition is helpful too.

5.   Reward yourself- If you are making progress with your morning workouts, don't forget to reward yourself. Watch that latest blockbuster movie or buy yourself a ticket to a game of basketball featuring your favorite team.

6.   Pay attention to nutrition- If you are going to be working out religiously every morning, you do have to pay adequate attention to your nutrition or you will feel inordinately fatigued through the day. Make it a point to have a wholesome breakfast after a vigorous workout so that you are able to fully capitalize on the hard work put in by you.

It is often said that the best things in life are free. You could say that about morning exercise, though it might not be entirely free of cost. But in terms of the benefits it provides you, it might as well as be considered that. There really is no price that you can put on good health, longevity and a sterling quality of life. Truly, early morning exercise bestows nothing less than the very gift of life.